The Sad Stays

Ashley Lumpkin

A Memoir

Greensboro / 2024
Scuppernong Editions

THE SAD STAYS

So. Picture this: A teacher/poet sits at the counter of her favorite bookstore for two or so hours on a Sunday. Intermittently, her friends and other bookstore patrons offer to buy her a glass of wine and ask what she's working on.

Sometimes she says a poem. Sometimes an essay. Sometimes, she just laughs and shakes her head. Eventually, she settles on the word *memoir* with vague hand gestures and questioning intonation, knowing that coming to terms with what it is will be as difficult as discussing what it's about.

In 2012, after years of struggling with my mental health, I was diagnosed with Bipolar II Disorder. The defining symptoms began presenting themselves nearly five years before I sought any type of medical professional, preferring a mix between self-determination and praying the crazy away. Even with a diagnosis, I was resistant to most forms of what people called *help*—resistant even to the idea of what it meant to get better. This was long before the era of *"it's ok not to be ok."* Everything I knew about the illness came from wildly unflattering film and TV portrayals of people unable to keep it together. They couldn't hold jobs or build families—not for long anyway—they were unstable, untrustworthy, generally burdensome—the antithesis of the person I wanted to be. Even casually, apart from a clinical diagnosis, the phrase *"she's so bipolar"* became a shocking blow. It meant moody. Unreliable. Too much to handle. Meant, if nothing else, I should hide—keep the diagnosis to myself.

Over the course of the next several years, through many therapists, one Christian counselor, and a handful of psychiatrists, that diagnosis morphed through the many forms of BiPD, with a brief detour into an ADHD seasonal affective disorder combo pack, until finally landing at a (slightly) less daunting declaration of a run-of-the-mill depression and anxiety blend. Sometimes the names felt useful—a bridge toward getting the right kind of help. Sometimes the names were further proof that help would always be just out of reach. The handful of people that were *"in the know"* approached the labels with varying degrees of shock and seriousness. For some, they were answers to a question they hadn't been allowed to ask; for others, they were an understandable reason to walk away.

What follows is an exploration of living with bipolar disorder, or whatever the correct label is (or was) for my particular brand of emotional unrest.

I am tempted at times to say the initial diagnosis was wrong. Symptoms change. The DSM eventually gets revised. My ego, at times, got in the way of being honest about all I was going through. The gratitude from the other side of an episode clouds the memory of walking through it. I am tempted at times to hold up the word *"better"* as proof that there is no longer a threat that I'll turn into one of those characters I watched fearfully on so many screens. Instead, I say, *"faithfully managed,"* and try my best not to live on edge.

A memoir, they tell me, is a historical account, and that I should be concerned mostly with sharing the facts. The truth is, sometimes the facts are lost in the haze of the illness itself. Memory can change the shape of a room, fade colors, blend even time and space. So, no, I cannot promise this is exactly how it happened, but you can trust this is exactly how it felt.

She asks me if my friends trust me. As if it's some sort of *yes* or *no* question. Like it's a thing people can just do or not do. Even though I can tell by looking around this place that it's not the way she thinks. Everything about the room seems to be the work of someone intent upon making a perfectly common space seem unique. It's one of several in a building that itself belongs to a complex of identical, red-bricked buildings in an otherwise remote part of town. There's a dentist, a law office, one for rent, a chiropractor's clinic, and this place—which seems to be fighting the surrounding scent of sterility with those plug-ins that try to convince the nose it's in a meadow and not seeing a therapist.

The receptionist at the desk was neither cold nor familiar. The chairs in the waiting room neither comfortable nor unpleasant. And the lights in the office were neither on nor off. I mean the overhead lights that some architect or engineer installed at the beginning of all this office space—those are off. But the lamp on the side table between her chair and the couch on which I am seated is on. It seems like one of those lamps where the brightness changes depending on how many times you pull the string, but there is no visible string. Either way, it appears she made a conscious choice to make the room this dim.

On the table, a flimsy little book is open with a clip-on book light attached—still on, as though this appointment snuck up on her somehow. She seems like the kind of person that would have a plant in the corner. Instead, there's an open space begging for some kind of art installation— an enormous glass piece of winding curves that could reflect the on and not-on lights, but there is no time for curves. That would involve learning to sculpt or handle something with intention. There was that week after my painting obsession where I made little figurines from plastic straws, or the dream that pops up from time to time about becoming a master ceramicist, which seems like it could be the perfect lead-in to a promising career with molten glass, but how can I focus on a new career path when I'm supposed to be answering a question.

Yes. They trust me.
Which is not entirely true. Which I know she knows because of the way she cocks her head to the side and clicks on the retractable pen that had, up until then, been held in its cage.

Not like, to do things, I guess. I cancel plans a lot.
Which is also not entirely true. I don't know that I cancel the plans that I actually make—but the ones that I make when even at that second, I have zero intention of following through—those I flake on all the time. Like this appointment, for example. Weeks ago, I called Dr. No Lights' office with every intention of cancelling even as I was selecting the date, but this morning I realized I'd missed the window in which I could do so without having to pay for it anyway. Maybe if my friends charged in advance—like little Chuck E. Cheese tokens they could cash in for returned text messages and dinners out—I'd be less apt to pretend like something came up, but it's not about doing things, I think.

I mean, the night Mer flipped her entire body over the stair railing of the apartment we all sort of lived in but didn't pay rent for, she knew, without asking that I wouldn't tell anyone the things that really made her run from the room. And isn't that more important than being trusted for something as silly as follow-through?

But like—me—they trust me.
I mean I'm not the type of person that's going to actually take up glass blowing on a whim anymore, but once, when London mentioned tossing the ball around with her brother, not an hour later I bought us each a glove, bat, a few balls, and four bean bags large enough to stand in for bases. And yes, I've always been good with words, but doesn't it seem nearly impossible to convince thirteen or so strangers that the weird girl they've seen around campus but don't ever really remember talking to is absolutely right about their need to ignore their studies during finals' week to go outside and play a little ball?

She doesn't seem impressed. She leans in to remind me that, in one of our previous sessions, I suggested that my spending habits got out of hand in college. But whose aren't under close examination? And what is money when stacked up against a friend's need to feel a little calmer on a Saturday afternoon, even if it means not eating the next week? Like, what is the point of money, if not to recommission the architect who designed this building to come in and re-do all the light fixtures? And would that be altogether strange of me to offer? To brainstorm? To plan? Can I write my therapist a check to give to the building manager on my behalf? To keep her from being the kind of person who relies on a book light for atmosphere?

What I'm saying is they can count on me—you know—when it matters. Except for the times they cannot. But I'm not the type of person that talks about that. Because who wants to hear all that anyway? So what if six months ago, I quit my job and told everyone that it was to follow my dreams? So what if my passions turned out to be not showering and staying in bed? But before all that. When Angie needed a hug from her boyfriend who lived five and a half states away, she hopped in my car and rode all thirteen hours with no other questions asked. Did Dr. Needs New Lamps have a friend she could count on like that? To go hungry to keep her fed?

She says something about impulsivity. About believing that I held things together. About the way my ego swings from hill to valley with little to no explanation. About lights flickering behind my eyes and some off-kilter hormones controlling the switch. She is the fourth in a line of therapists who believe there is something more wrong with me than not understanding why I can't seem to start sleeping—or stop—when I want to. But who does that? Start calling the inside of their own head by some other, doctor-prescribed name? Especially this doctor, who claims to have the power of diagnosis, but not the power to remember an appointment in time to put her leisure reading away.

But what does that matter? If they can depend on me? She asks if I remember the last time I trusted myself.

But isn't that the problem? That I always trust myself? To know the right answer? To be the right answer? Be the one with the baseball gloves in the backseat who will drive you up the coast without anyone knowing? Playing catch in a coffee shop a sunrise away because someone cashed in all their tokens? And it's not all bad. Like that's a thing your mind can just be or not be. If it were, wouldn't I have just flipped that switch a long time ago?

She looks around the room—the box of Kleenex by the lamp, the empty space in the corner, the wall clock positioned above and behind my head. She waits for me to answer. To say something worth writing down. To mention anything she might suggest we work on in our next session. Even though I know there will be no next one. I know that Dr. Dim Room is on the verge of a diagnosis—or at least of positing theories for all the noise inside my head—and isn't that where most relationships end? When you insist upon giving them a label?

Trust myself? Is that something I can just do? Or not do?
She cocks her head to the side and makes a few notes on her legal pad. She tells me we are out of time, picks the book up from the side table. She undoes the clasp of the booklight and sets it down on the table. She suggests I read the pages in the book that she's flagged—that we'll talk through my response the following week. I wonder if she knows she doesn't have any tokens.

Don't forget to turn that light off.

CLIENT INTAKE FORM

This form is used to collect information about new clients and is for internal purposes only. The information you provide is confidential and will be treated accordingly.

REASONS FOR VISIT

What are the problems for which you are seeking help?

Do you know what a poetry slam is? It's like the bad poetry readings that you see on TV, except…the poems are good, and no one is snapping their fingers because it's not 1952, and who owns a beret? Anyway. Imagine that. Except after you recite your poem, there are five random people giving Olympic style scores to whatever it is you just talked about. 5.2, 7.6, 8.3. Whatever. I do that. Compete in them. And now I'm on a team, and we just got back from our first big festival, and I have not been able to sleep. One night of no sleep is no big deal, I know, but I was only getting a few hours a night at the festival itself, and now I get even less than that.

We came in fifth place at the festival. Highest ranking in quite a few years. I don't need help for that, I'm just saying—the not sleeping might have helped. Now though, I'd like to be able to crash.

Current Symptoms: (check all that apply)

☒ Racing thoughts	☒ Fatigue	☐ Excessive energy	☐ Depressed mood
☐ Suspiciousness	☐ Hallucinations	☐ Impulsivity	☐ Loss of interest
☐ Avoidance	☐ Forgetfulness	☐ Change in appetite	☐ Crying spell
☐ Anxiety Attacks	☐ Excessive Guilt	☐ Excessive worry	☐ Increased irritiability
☒ Sleep pattern disturbance	☐ Unable to enjoy activities	☐ Increased risky behavior	☒ Decreased need for sleep

June 2010

SOME TERMS FOR BIPOLAR STUDIES

episode	is someone watching? can they change the channel?
bipolar	(slang) emotional, indecisive, impulsive, flaky
dsm 5	an allegorical text on things not to say to your therapist
infertility	a gift
genetic	dad's mom went missing sometimes too, when the crying got too bad
hallucination	(see memory)
memory	(see hallucination)
depression	that one time, waking up hungry and sore—hadn't left the bed in six days
diagnosis	the word all of your exes scream as they walk out the door
insomnia	an ancient custom, believed to summon god
roller coaster	a lazy metaphor, a thrill ride with a safety net
mania	that one time, hungry and sore—hadn't found sleep in six days
trauma	another name for Tuesday
prayer	an honest conversation with the most quiet voice inside your head
symptom	the start of every story you have for breaking the ice
sleep	an ancient custom, believed to summon god
fear	potentially an indication that you are headed toward an even state; alternately, the first sign of worse to come
disorder(ed)	the way it's always been
normal	two pills a day, reaching toward a forgotten hallucination

MONTAGE

EXT. DORM PARKING LOT—NIGHT

Ashley and four other young women stand near her fairly new car. She
is on the banking app on her phone; her negative balance is visible.
We see her pull up a messaging app. She texts, "Lights about to be
cut off. Can I borrow some cash?" to an unknown contact.

Laughing, she gets into the driver's seat of the car.

INT. CAR PARKED IN DORM PARKING LOT—MOMENTS LATER

Ashley pulls the phone out of her pocket and reads a notification.
She smiles and turns the keys in the ignition.

EXT. HIGHWAY / NEW YORK STATE LINE—LATER THAT NIGHT

We see the car driving past a "Welcome to New York" sign.

EXT. STRANGER'S BACKYARD—NIGHT

Ashley is making out with a stranger (as few discernable features
as possible) while a group crowds around cheering. She is only 5
shots into a pass-out-drunk night, but she is in love with being the
center of attention.

INT. CAR PARKED IN A WALMART PARKING LOT—DAY

Ashley is making out with a different stranger in the back seat
of her car. Walmart customers can be seen peering in through the
windshield, some with voyeuristic amusement, others with disgust.

INT. ASHLEY'S APARTMENT—NIGHT

Ashley stands at the kitchen counter, laughing while haphazardly
tossing envelopes into the trash can. They are from various credit
card companies, debt collectors, and utility companies—all with
"Past Due" or "Final Notice" stamped on the front. Last in the pile
is an eviction notice. She tosses this into the garbage too.

INT. VARIOUS LOCATIONS—DAY / NIGHT

We see Ashley on her knees and sobbing in

...her apartment

...her best friend's kitchen

...on the dance floor in a night club

...backstage in the wings of a small theatre

INT. STAGE—NIGHT / MOMENTS LATER

Ashley walks to a microphone that is set center stage in a 150-seat theatre. Every seat is filled, and the room is silent. She begins speaking to the crowd without a moment of hesitation. She is in love with being the center of attention.

EXT. PARKING LOT—NIGHT

It is raining. Ashley sits on the ground, near her car. She is shaking uncontrollably. It is unclear if she is laughing or crying.

END MONTAGE.

VAN GOGH STEPS INTO THE KITCHEN
AND SHARPENS MY KNIVES

Listen kid
        he says,
taking in the sunflowers standing tall in the vase

*We get it. You're a preacher's kid with a silver tongue
and a love of drafting self-portraits. Who among us isn't?*

Teacher?
        check.
Broken?
        check.

*Too drunk with the sadness to know your reflection? I
would call you a cliché at this point, but how would that
further the language? I mean, you got the chops kid, but
are you really committed? What would you give to know it
was possible to change the world? What if the only world
that changed was the one inside your own head?*

He puts a hand on each of my shoulders, commands
the stars in my eyes to swift understanding. He spins on
his heels and leaves the room, pulling at his good ear
as he goes.

RESEARCH
(Erasure 1)

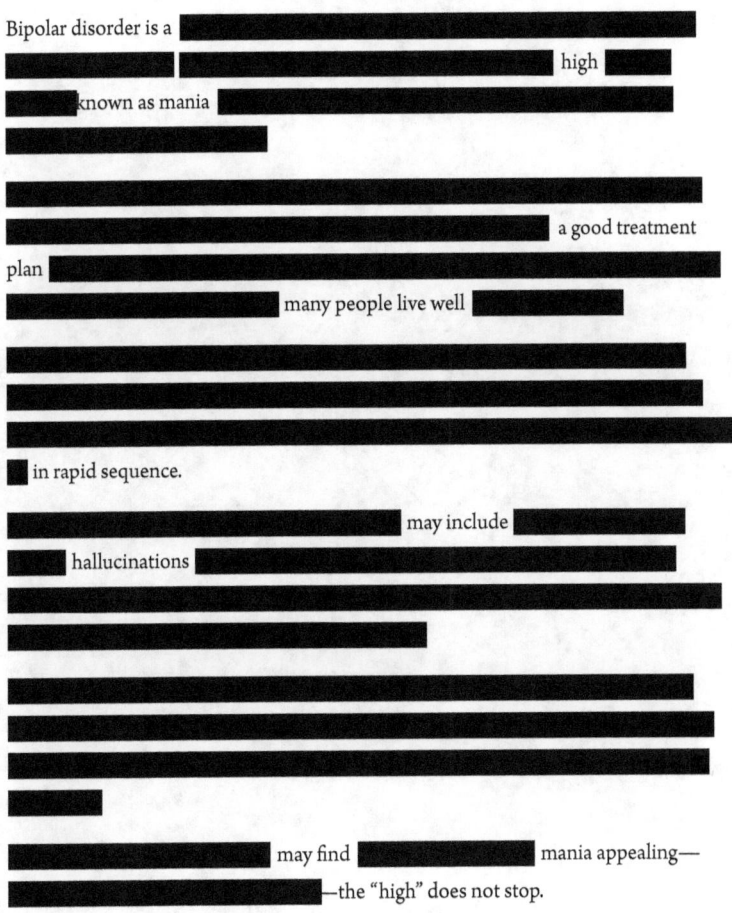

Bipolar disorder is a ▮▮▮▮▮▮▮▮▮▮▮▮▮▮▮▮▮▮▮▮▮▮▮▮▮
▮▮▮▮▮▮▮▮▮ ▮▮▮▮▮▮▮▮▮▮▮▮▮▮▮▮▮▮▮▮▮▮▮ high ▮▮▮
▮▮▮ known as mania ▮▮▮▮▮▮▮▮▮▮▮▮▮▮▮▮▮▮▮▮
▮▮▮▮▮▮▮▮▮▮▮▮

▮▮▮▮▮▮▮▮▮▮▮▮▮▮▮▮▮▮▮▮▮▮▮▮▮▮▮▮▮▮▮▮
▮▮▮▮▮▮▮▮▮▮▮▮▮▮▮▮▮▮▮▮▮▮▮▮ a good treatment
plan ▮▮▮▮▮▮▮▮▮▮▮▮▮▮▮▮▮▮▮▮▮▮▮▮▮▮▮▮▮▮
▮▮▮▮▮▮▮▮ many people live well ▮▮▮▮▮▮▮▮

▮▮▮▮▮▮▮▮▮▮▮▮▮▮▮▮▮▮▮▮▮▮▮▮▮▮▮▮▮▮
▮▮▮▮▮▮▮▮▮▮▮▮▮▮▮▮▮▮▮▮▮▮▮▮▮▮▮▮▮▮
▮▮▮▮▮▮▮▮▮▮▮▮▮▮▮▮▮▮▮▮▮▮▮▮▮▮▮▮▮▮▮▮
▮ in rapid sequence.

▮▮▮▮▮▮▮▮▮▮▮▮▮▮▮▮▮▮▮▮▮ may include ▮▮▮▮▮▮
▮▮▮ hallucinations ▮▮▮▮▮▮▮▮▮▮▮▮▮▮▮▮▮▮▮▮▮▮
▮▮▮▮▮▮▮▮▮▮▮▮▮▮▮▮▮▮▮▮▮▮▮▮▮▮▮▮▮▮▮
▮▮▮▮▮▮▮▮▮▮▮▮▮▮▮

▮▮▮▮▮▮▮▮▮▮▮▮▮▮▮▮▮▮▮▮▮▮▮▮▮▮▮▮▮
▮▮▮▮▮▮▮▮▮▮▮▮▮▮▮▮▮▮▮▮▮▮▮▮▮▮▮▮▮▮▮
▮▮▮▮▮▮▮▮▮▮▮▮▮▮▮▮▮▮▮▮▮▮▮▮▮▮▮▮▮▮
▮▮▮▮

▮▮▮▮▮▮▮▮▮▮▮▮▮▮▮ may find ▮▮▮▮▮▮▮▮▮ mania appealing—
▮▮▮▮▮▮▮▮▮▮▮▮▮▮▮▮▮—the "high" does not stop.

And you hate more than anything to be a cliché, but the conversations you've heard on all those bad TV shows where the girl who is a little too honest for the main character's liking, after kissing the best friend instead of him, has to *"come down"* with some mental illness that absolutely must be medicated—and the music swells while she sobs and shouts, *"I just don't feel like myself anymore."* And the scene is ridiculous, but your doctor describes every aspect of what you call personality as a symptom of this new disorder—every road trip, doubledare, shopping spree, nightmare, breakdown, as something that could have been medicated away, but then who would you be? Even the parts that have almost killed you were the things worth writing poetry about, and isn't that who you are too? Aren't the poems what make you possible? If all of it is suddenly stripped away, is the thing that's left actually you? Where is the line that separates what you see in the mirror from the thing they call your disease?

Because let's face it, even if you don't take the pills, your mind doesn't automatically dissolve into panic. It's not all liquor and sad guitars, hunched over a notebook on a Thursday night. It is those things too, sometimes, but mostly it's just Friday at the bar: And your best friend has finally gotten the dollar jukebox to play that song you danced to that one night on a dare, mostly because she didn't believe you when you explained how you'd perfected this seated swaying, which gave the illusion that you could really dance if only you would commit to putting in effort, when, in reality, if you actually stood, it would all devolve into something you'd learned in a high school modern dance class, which is absolutely not what Cash Money took over the 99s and 2000s for. And the two of you are laughing as you race to the dance floor, so hard you think you might fall over. And you try to make the near falling a part of the dance, but you're both too clumsy and uncoordinated for that and just end up grabbing each other by the shoulders and twirling around, throwing your heads back to laugh into the ceiling, which feels so much like the sky.

In eighth grade you learned about Orion's Belt, among a host of other constellations—your homework to stand outside each night and attempt to ascribe the right names to heaven. You learned about the Star Registry and consider naming a star after yourself. Maybe one for each of your siblings and closest friends too. You could populate an entire galaxy with the names that were most meaningful, or even ones that just sounded cool until every sparkling thing in the firmament somehow belonged to you. As it was, Orion's belt was the only one you could really see, cocking your ear to shoulder and picking any three stars in alignment to be the belt of the hunter shooting his arrows at the north star.

And the boys at the other side of the bar who tried to send you drinks earlier in the evening see you spinning, and you see the question marks on their faces, wondering whose dime you're having that kind of good time on, and that thought sends you deeper into your belly to find the kind of laugh you haven't had in a long time. But you can't remember it. And that—the lack of memory—for just a moment, is enough to hollow your insides and send you spiraling into yourself and all the other things you haven't done for too long now. And just like that, knowing you haven't really laughed in years, and believing it will be years before you laugh that way again, takes you from spinning top to lead weight—even while your friend is still dancing. And so are you. In the way that your feet are still moving, even though there is no ground beneath you.

And eighth grade, one of your doctors will say later, is too young for a true depressive episode, though not too young to be depressed—to lay on the grass and contemplate what it means to be the target of Orion's arrow-hunted star, a celestial body under threat, a hidden constellation. How could you possibly want to medicate that kind of thinking away? Even if the grass was soaked from an afternoon rain, and your brothers had to convince you to come inside and stop all that weeping?

There are more reckless ways to spend this night. You could find another bar on the far side of another town and continue sleeping your way through the alphabet. You were almost onto O until you heard some idiot call the boy whose name you believed was Nick by another name, and discovered he'd gone by a shortened version of his last name since his final year in college, and of course last names don't count. You considered starting over again after a mishap of that proportion, but Franklin had been so hard to find that you almost started running door to door in your apartment complex, trying to find someone who met this very simple criterion.

But wouldn't that defeat the purpose? On a night when you had just been laughing, having a night that was not supposed to be a story to find some boy to pour all your hollow into? And not just some boy. A real Nick. Or Nelson. Ned. Nathaniel. Anyone who would think your request more humorous than strange. Anyone willing to become a brand-new star in this constellation.

And the boys on the side of the bar will not stop staring. And your best friend does not seem to notice that you've had that look in your eye for long enough now that she should start to get worried. And you think about starting your meds again as the song begins to fade. While you miss the night sky. And there is still no ground beneath you.

DIAGNOSIS

	YES	NO
Has there ever been a period of time where you were not your usual self? So much so that other people began to notice?	○	○
And were you more self-confident than usual?	○	○
With more energy than usual?	○	○
Have you ever felt good? About yourself?	○	○
Did you define yourself by the good that you felt? Were you ready to take on the world?	○	○
Did it get too confrontational?	○	○
Has there ever been a period of time where you were not your usual self, and were so irritable that you shouted at people or started fights or arguments?	○	○
Were they eloquent speeches?	○	○
Did your mind race?	○	○
Were you aware at all of which version of yourself you were fighting or racing against?	○	○
If you answered yes to more than one of these questions, did they occur within the same window of time?	○	○
Do you believe in time?	○	○
Do you remember yesterday?	○	○
Has there ever been a period of time where you wanted to hold on to yesterday so desperately you could not allow yourself to punctuate it with sleep?	○	○
Does sleep make a difference?	○	○

Is it overrated? ○ ○

Were you able to stare into the night sky and hear it whisper its infinite secrets? ○ ○

Did you try to explain this truth to your friends? ○ ○

Were they able to finally understand? ○ ○

Has there ever been a period of time when you were not your usual self, and you were much more talkative or spoke faster than usual? ○ ○

Were you so easily distracted by things around you that you had trouble concentrating or staying on track? ○ ○

Aren't you tired of the beaten path? ○ ○

Wouldn't they all be better off if they would just start listening to what you have to say? Even if it is the middle of the night? And they've heard all of this rambling before? And have asked you not to call this late unless it's an emergency and you were on your meds? ○ ○

Do you feel like you're always on? ○ ○

Is all of it just a performance? ○ ○

Are you ready to take a bow? ○ ○

In this version of the examination are you trying to pass or fail? ○ ○

BLOOD TEST

FADE IN:

EXT. CITY PARK—DAY

It's a crisp, clear, fall afternoon.

ASHLEY, an early-twenties Black woman, lies on her back on a park bench, staring into a cloudless sky. She has just left the outpatient clinic of a large hospital, visible in the background. Her best friend *RENEE*, an early-twenties Black woman, lies on the ground in front of her, scrolling through social media on a recently outdated smartphone.

Both are apprehensive, unsure of how to start the conversation.

                    RENEE
          You want to tell me what all of that was about?

                    ASHLEY
          Thanks for coming with. Needles and what not.

                    RENEE
          Unnecessary and what not. What was the point?
          Is the thing with the blood coming back again?

                    ASHLEY
          Thing with the blood? No. That's not a thing.

                    RENEE
          Then talk to me. C'mon. What are we doing here?

                    ASHLEY
          Just looking for a definitive answer.

                    RENEE
          Babe. We've talked about this. We've already
          reached *definitive*. Passed *definitive* really.
                    (Beat)
          You've gotta stop running to new doctors and
          accept that you really do have a thing.

                    ASHLEY
          Heard.
                    (Beat)
          It's just that other people have it so easy.

                    RENEE
What other people?

                    ASHLEY
Other people. The cancers and chickenpox.
Asthmatics or whomever.

                    RENEE
I'm pretty sure that those people don't have
it easy.

                    ASHLEY
You know that's not what I mean. Not easy.
Like, of course. And you know I have asthma.
Not breathing well obviously doesn't feel good
or whatever.

                    RENEE
I'm pretty sure you can't call them [sits up
and does air quotes] *the cancers* either.

                    ASHLEY
I'm pretty sure that anyone who does air quotes
in this decade can definitely kiss my ass.

                    (Beat)

It'd just be better to be sick or something,
I think.

*Renee stands to join Ashley on the bench. Ashley sits up and scoots,
so that her legs are now dangling off the edge. Renee sits, and
Ashley lies down, head in Renee's lap.*

                    RENEE
Well. You are sick. Also, chicken pox? Are you
comparing cancer to chicken pox? You can't
compare cancer and chicken pox.

                    ASHLEY
Obviously, I'm not comparing them. I'm just
saying a disease is a disease is all. That
having one people recognize would be better.

                    RENEE
I think it's better if you just start getting
used to this idea.

                    ASHLEY
I am getting used to it.

                    RENEE
So again.

                    (Beat)

Why are we here?

                    ASHLEY
To get a blood test.

                    RENEE
What kind of blood test?

                    ASHLEY
The kind that says if I'm sick or not.

                    RENEE
This kind of thing, babe, it's not in the blood.

                    ASHLEY
I know.

                    RENEE
Do you really? Then what was all that back
there then? All those symptoms? Did you make
that up—

                    ASHLEY
Not made up.

                    RENEE
You tried to say you were having heart
palpitations. I have literally never heard you
use the word palpitations before.

                    ASHLEY
Not made up.

                    (Beat)

Maybe I don't feel comfortable talking to you
about my palpitations. I mean, I can't even
talk to you about chicken pox.

                    RENEE
Did you make all that up just to make them do
some kind of blood draw?

                    (Beat)

This thing you've got...you know it doesn't
change anything right?

                    ASHLEY
Except now I'm not really me. Not the way I
think I am.

                    (Beat)

I feel normal. I feel like...like I feel
things. Like things are important to me. I feel
like if all that—the way a person thinks and
dreams and imagines and wants and wishes for
and needs—if all of that is somehow a symptom
of a disease, it should be kind enough to show
up in the bloodstream. *Yes, you've got it. No,
you don't*. Not so much of this speculation.

                    RENEE
Several people have already told you what this
is. I feel like I keep having to tell you that
we are well beyond speculation at this point.

                    ASHLEY
They've said likely.

                    RENEE
Ok. But *likely* from three different doctors
should resonate as a little more than just
likely. Why isn't that good enough?

                    ASHLEY
You'd think someone with a medical degree
would be able to give me some certainty. Tell
me if this thing is real.

                    RENEE
It's all real, babe.

                    ASHLEY
Yeah, but not the kind of real they give you
the good pills for.

                    RENEE
Well, they're going to give you pills. So, you'll
have that in common with the cancers at least.

*Both women erupt into laughter—subdued at first and then more
hysterical. Ashley comes to an upright position on the bench.
Still laughing, Renee takes her hand. After a moment, the laughter
subsides. Ashley looks into the distance. It is unclear whether she
is crying.*

                    RENEE
You'll take the meds. You'll see the shrinks.
We'll get a routine. And you'll get better.

                    ASHLEY
Mm.

                    RENEE
Or you'll go off the deep end, and we will
fight like hell to bring you back.

                    ASHLEY
Mm.

                    RENEE
I promise. We will always bring you back.

                                        FADE OUT.

In the dream, she is sixteen years old. A little shorter than me. Definitely prettier. Not quite the same sense of style, but the exact humor—though in the dream she is rarely laughing. Barely cracks a smile.

I appear in the hallway. I don't have a grasp on the size and shape of the building. In the dream, I walk through no doors. I can hear my mother praying in the voice she normally reserves for church—the one that is part singer, part auctioneer—to let god know she means business. When we were much younger, playing make-believe church, I am tempted to say it's a voice we mimicked, though I can't quite picture us mocking our mother or remember the game itself.

If I am honest, I only have three memories of my sister. The rest is imagination, filling in the gaps.

Age nine and six, the two of us tucked beneath the winter coats in the hall closet after school. We are convinced it is our secret hiding place without once questioning the snacks that awaited us every afternoon when we returned from school. And she has the same teacher I had in first grade, so I give all sorts of insider secrets: become best friends with the best drawer in class, and you won't have to illustrate your own stories; pay attention to the voices when she reads *Charlotte's Web*, because at the end, she will need someone to read, because she starts to cry and cannot go on, and she will definitely call on you if you can sound like her version of Templeton. But on this day, we are discussing none of that—just laughing about the bus ride home. How all of us, even the shy kids at the front, were so loud that Ms. D pulled over and glared at us, refusing to move until we were stilled into silence.

Age fourteen and eleven, in our grandmother's living room, with music our parents did not approve of blaring loudly from our cousin's CD player. This kind of music was the reason our father pulled us off the school bus—the day he heard us singing *Candy Rain* at the top of our lungs. And for all of that sheltering he still sends us South to our extended family to connect with the parts of ourselves he left home to forget. My favorite aunt is so proud that she was able to purchase the player and a few CDs. She thinks it's hysterical that you both go to that fancy art school, but somehow have no taste in music.

Even funnier that you will only nod along to the songs because neither of you can dance.

And then, five years later, in the halls of the hospital, begging god to send her soul back to her body, even though she hated it—rail thin with calloused knuckles, enamel eroding from her teeth.

This is the memory that folds itself into all the nightmares:

Our younger brother sits next to the bed, not quite holding her hand. His eyes are fixed on a flake of chipped paint above the chorus of monitors, taking in the beeps and clicks made by the machines. His right foot plays an invisible bass drum, his left shakes with a much less rhythmic grief. Our older brother also sways to a music no one in the room can hear, his head bowed as though praying, but really more as an excuse to let a few tears fall. He stands in the corner near the window, his hand on our mother's shoulder as she kneels.

In some versions of the dream, she is talking and trying to smile. In others, the pain she is in shocks her into quiet. Every version is hard to explain. It is practically impossible to contend with the truth: I did not have a baby sister. She is a figment of my imagination—an apparition my mind created to protect itself—breaking from reality at least three times and leaving me to fill in the rest. My sister was smart. Thoughtful. A brilliant pianist. Funny. In a pain she never admitted, and died when I was nineteen years old.

In the dream, the whole room glows, though there's no discernable source of light. The volume of the beeping rattles the walls, though somehow the entire room is silent. My brothers come to attention, screaming for help and saying no words. A nurse appears. Goes. Appears again. He pulls at the cords and presses buttons. He does not touch her—not even once. We are all shouting. We are all sobbing. I cannot hear a sound.

There are days I still beat myself up for not having done more to save her—then beat myself up again for not remembering she never was. I have spent countless hours researching false memories and the disorders of which they are symptomatic. Find myself wishing I had more of those memories, even though it means welcoming the psychosis. I imagine what it would be like to not have to grieve the apparition, but to sit with her now in my own coat closet to laugh about our days. We'd have popcorn and wine and tell problematic jokes where my illness was both straight man and punchline. Perhaps I'd be too far down the rabbit hole to care that this only existed in my mind.

In the dream, the room shifts—goes stark white. I am seated alone at her bedside, praying and humming *Candy Rain* as a sort of clumsy goodbye. And then, at the last moment, she does what she did not.

In the dream, I call her by name, and just once, she opens her eyes.

HYMN 245
(Erasure 2)

PRAYER

O Lord, My God, I Thirst For You

245

Text: Anthony Robertson, 2010. Music: 'Kingsfold' traditional English. Setting: Ralph Vaughan Williams, 1906.
copyright: music and setting public domain. Words: Copyright 2010, Anthony Robertson. These lyrics may be
freely reproduced or published for Christian worship, provided they are not altered, and this notice is
on each copy. All other rights reserved. This score is a part of the Open Hymnal Project, 2013 Revision.

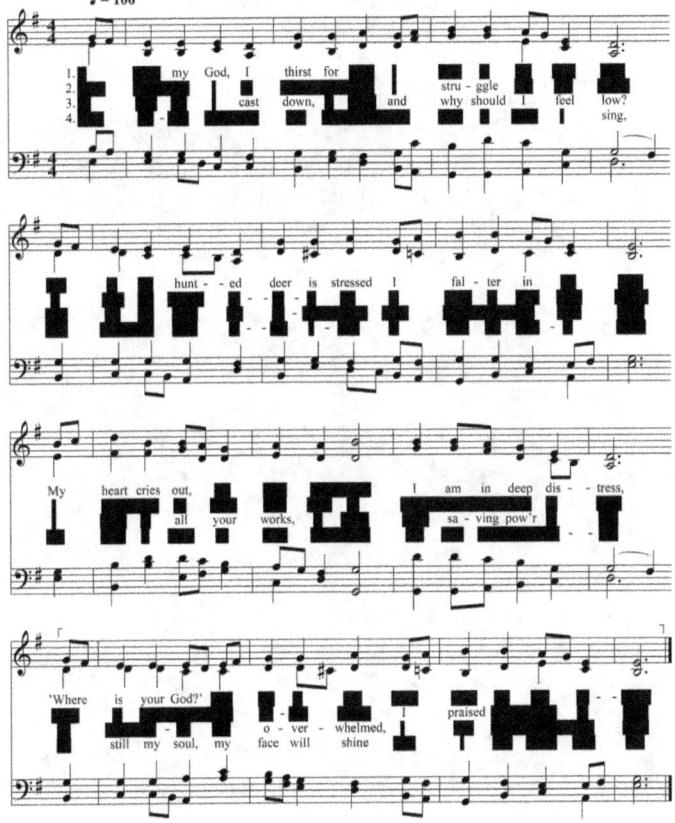

Ps 42:1-11, Job 13:15-16, Is 50:8-11, Lam 3:24, Rom 8:35-39

8 6 8 6 8 6 8 6

where is your god / my heart cries out
in deep distress / and cast down

i falter as hunted / deer is distressed
i thirst / for saving power

i am my god / my face will shine
still my soul / overwhelmed in struggle

i sing a praise / to all my works
my hope set / why should i feel low

Bipolar disorder is ███████████████████████████
███
███████ years—without symptoms. ███████████████
███████████████

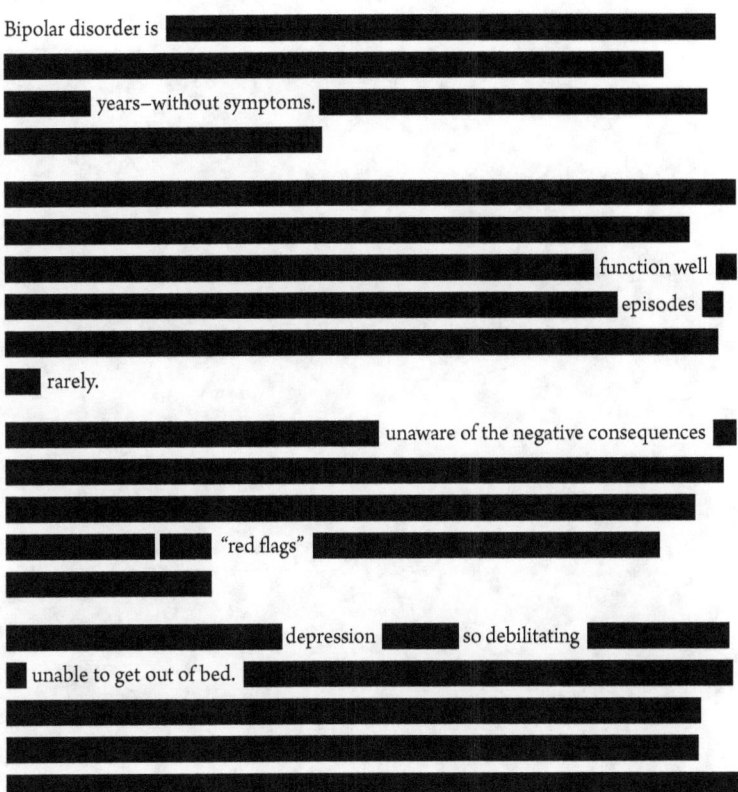

███
███████████████████████████████████████
███████████████████████████████████████ function well █
███████████████████████████████████████ episodes █
███
█ rarely.

███████████████████████████████ unaware of the negative consequences █
███
███████████████████████████████████████
███████████ ███ "red flags" ███████████████████
███████████████

███████████████████████ depression ██████ so debilitating █████████
█ unable to get out of bed. ███████████████████████
███████████████████████████████████
███████████████████████████████████
███

SIX FLAGS OVER THIS DEPRESSION

fun fact about living with bipolar disorder
for some of us it is a disease we grow out of

research says, if you go two years without mania
it is probable to not have a manic episode again

it has been one year and ten months
since the last time i was so happy i almost died
the thrill ride of my theme park existence
found an even piece of track i hope it rides out on

my friend thinks i should throw a party, and now
my calendar a countdown to an eerie holiday i shouldn't really celebrate
because most folks don't know that i have an illness
most folks see the symptoms and call it a good time:

say road trip shopping spree sexual liberation
suicidal while singing on a bridge in arkansas

and then what if indeed i do throw a party
and my mind forgets to cut off the music

the calendar now becomes a reminder
of the last time i had a decent night's sleep
or a hold on my spending, or control of my body
the last i smiled and wasn't dying

i'd be caught in this two-step i started myself
all because i allowed one moment of hope
so maybe i will stop with the countdown
maybe i will just write a poem.

fun fact about bipolar disorder
manic episodes can begin as creativity

the mania stands to declare itself
says, i am a good idea
that this idea is worthy of a stage

that being on stage can change the world
and suddenly it's not a poem any more
it's a book a movie a platform a podcast

it's the entire world in my room at midnight hanging on to my every word
like a group of children watching a commercial for the newest amusement park
and what is the fun of an amusement park if not to see how close you can get
to death but somehow walk away smiling

and once
a friend described being bipolar as something like a roller coaster
like highs and lows and a little fear
but something we all survive

but what if you came to the amusement park
and they had done away with every safety harness
people falling from the top of each hill as you waited in line

is the amusement park still fun
knowing there's a fifty percent chance you'll jump once you get on the ride
knowing that it takes two years to earn your spot out of the line
and talking about the possibility of leaving is a sure sign you'll be stuck there

fun fact about having bipolar disorder
the fun part is the most dangerous

and i haven't been manic in almost two years
except maybe now
that i want to write about it

FIFTEEN PERCENT

FADE IN:

INT. APARTMENT BATHROOM—NIGHT

The shower has been running for quite a while now. Everything is steamy and damp. The rug has been pushed to the far side of the bathroom. ASHLEY sits, her back to the wall, eyes darting back and forth, with an otherwise blank stare. We hear ALEX, a late twenties Black man, in the background. He is very clearly having an angry conversation with someone on the phone, but we cannot make out what he says.

                    ASHLEY
          (whispering)
          He's not wrong.
          He's not wrong.
          He's not wrong.
          He's not wrong.

                                             CUT TO:

INT. BEDROOM—CONTINIOUS

ALEX is pacing in the dark with his phone to his ear.

                    ALEX
          I know people change, Mom! Of course she's
          allowed to change! She's always changing. At
          this point, no two days are the same.

BACK TO SCENE

ASHLEY continues to mouth inaudibly as a voice over plays.

                    ASHLEY (V.O.)
          I cannot help that I am selfish. I think a lot
          about what that means. I wanted for a long
          time to get a narcissism diagnosis, because
          then at least I could point at another disease
          to blame, but no such luck for me. Even when
          I try, really try, to not be so selfish—
          there's a part of me that hopes he notices the
          selflessness and offers a bit of praise.

INTERCUT BETWEEN BEDROOM AND BATHROOM.

ALEX is inaudible, but increasingly upset.

ASHLEY (V.O.)
He can't want a child with that. He can't
assume the selfish will disappear just because
there's a baby involved. And is it selfish?
To not want a baby? Even without a so-called
reason, how does anyone go about changing the
things they desire? If I knew how to do that,
I could fix a laundry list of the world's
problems, but then of course I'd be far too
busy to be able to raise a child. But it's not
desire. I have a reason. Why doesn't he know I
would be a terrible mother? And if he cannot
see that, what other things can he not see?

And I've heard people say something will come
over me. That I will be overcome with a love
for the kid that changes me. Consumes me. Are
we certain that is even a good thing? What
is the difference between consumption and
unhealthy hyper-fixation? What if I'm too in
love with her voice to ever let her sleep?

Love was supposed to make me more willing to
sacrifice for him, and I can barely remember
to make sure the water he likes stays in our
fridge. What if he's waiting for the version
of me that is transformed? What if I am
incapable of being radically transformed?

They take children from mothers like that.
Mothers like that don't remember to make their
kids breakfast. Or wash them. They don't
remember to pray. Or take their meds. Or go to
work. They have to be told to hold the baby.
What if I never want to hold the baby? Feed
her? Change her? What if I can't convince
myself she's worth even getting out of bed? He
can't want that. Not a baby with me. Certainly
not my baby.

Three out of every twenty children born to a
mother with bipolar disorder wind up having
the disorder themselves. How can he take care
of me and a baby that will definitely be one
of the three?

And it doesn't even start when they are
little. He will be able to handle the first
two decades, even if I am on the floor. She'll
be smart and funny, and he will love her so
much that nothing will seem like a warning
sign. So, the first real blow-out will feel
like a surprise when he thinks he's all done

with the raising and bail outs and super-dad
stuff. Hasn't it been like that with my own
father? What if nothing skips a generation?
What else will bubble up in the blood?

It's all too much. I am already always too
much. No one stays with a person like that, no
matter how selfish it may seem to walk away.
And how can I be expected to take care of his
child when he eventually leaves?

                                          FADE TO:

ALEX is seated on the floor with his back to the wall. Spent.

                    ALEX
          I know, Mom. She isn't wrong.

I start the day with Red Bull and cigarettes, drafting Facebook statuses I will not post. My friends all think I've given up smoking because I have this crippling asthma. Really, all I've found is a better brand of e-cigarette. Some say the thought behind e-cigarettes is that they are somehow not bad for the lungs, but tell that to the cough this morning when I cannot catch my breath. I know the refusal to give up smoking is a sign I am functionally suicidal again. I should probably call my therapist, or at least a doctor to prescribe an inhaler until this wave of depression passes.

I think about my depression the same way atheists think about god— not much really, until a fanatic won't get out of their face. These days my depression won't get out of my face. It's the elephant in every room I enter until I become my own circus. I would call myself the ringmaster, if it weren't for this damn trapeze. I think about falling and hanging limp in the dark for days on end with no one to catch me, all of which I type into the status bar, but it reads too much like a cry for help. And isn't my partner on the trapeze just supposed to be there? Even at 3 a.m., when it's me and the Internet, reading an article about popcorn lung, a result of the chemicals in e-cigarettes that are also found in popcorn butter.

I think of the movie they will make of my life if I finally decide it's too hard to be here, my friends sitting in a crowded theatre, crying and chewing popcorn. And that is a little coincidence. And aren't those sorts of things beautiful? And aren't the beautiful things supposed to make me want to stay here?

Being functionally suicidal means I still go to work. Still go to church. Drive down the highway too fast with the windows down, hoping the cold will settle in my throat, and then, maybe pneumonia. Maybe I only take smoke breaks on the days I leave my inhaler at home on the dresser. Or maybe, I just stop calling my mother, the only woman who still prays for me. Who believes a real encounter with god is the only way depression passes.

I think about my depression the same way fanatics think about god—not much really, until someone they love is about to die. She posts scriptures on Facebook before she sleeps and prays they will swing to the top of my newsfeed, when nothing else too positive is coming down the line.

Being functionally suicidal means I don't want to die, I'm just not all that interested in trying to stay here either. It's like my life is a C-minus movie, with a rising star and ambiguous plot line that the studio hopes will do well but won't really get behind. It's like they know the only draw will be the tragic ending, a surprise fall, a snapped trapeze in a Three-Ring Circus with no ringmaster—a mother waiting in the ticket line trying to bring a little god in.

I think about my depression the same way I think about god. How it's the biggest thing in the room—even if no one sees it—whose existence is not predicated upon anyone's belief, and whether or not I bow to it feels like the only choice. Being functionally suicidal means each day is a choice. Each day is a fight. Every day a victory. Even if it feels like defeat.

CLIENT INTAKE FORM

This form is used to collect information about new clients and is for internal purposes only. The information you provide is confidential and will be treated accordingly.

REASONS FOR VISIT

What are the problems for which you are seeking help?

I've been at this teaching thing for years now, and every August sends me into overdrive. It's my favorite part of the calendar year—when the best version of me still feels possible. Hyper-productive. Hyper-focused. Unit plans. Classroom layout. New materials. All from scratch. All aimed at the good the new school year will bring.

Not this year, though. For some reason. Not yet. Teachers are supposed to return to school in a week, and I cannot make myself get out of bed. Can't get excited. Can't get motivated, and I have no idea how to jump start it.

They don't deserve that. My students, I mean. I haven't even met them all yet, and I'm already letting them down.

Current Symptoms: (check all that apply)

☐ Racing thoughts	☐ Fatigue	☐ Excessive energy	☒ Depressed mood
☐ Suspiciousness	☐ Hallucinations	☐ Impulsivity	☒ Loss of interest
☒ Avoidance	☐ Forgetfulness	☒ Change in appetite	☒ Crying spell
☐ Anxiety Attacks	☒ Excessive Guilt	☒ Excessive worry	☐ Increased irritiability
☐ Sleep pattern disturbance	☒ Unable to enjoy activities	☐ Increased risky behavior	☐ Decreased need for sleep

August 2013

The line in the sand of every diagnosis is its interference with day-to-day life. And it's not a sign of paranoia anymore to discuss the function of capitalism or its ability to force us into defining ourselves solely as profitable bodies.

What I mean is: Everyone hates getting out of bed in the morning. You get pills when you stop going to work. Or go, but can't quite seem to perform. Seem to position yourself between the door and the window, so in case of emergency you'll be able to respond. Are more obsessed with staying in position than doing the job you were paid to do, which had something to do with mathematics just a few years ago. But it's not enough to just teach anymore. The scope of the job has expanded, right? Not just algebra these days. You've got to teach the kids about hygiene and character as well— how to conform to fit into the machine, while nurturing any inner spark that's bright enough in them to rage against it. And then we plan for the emergency. Know where all the exits are. The escape routes. The places to gather. And this is what keeps me up at night. That somewhere, someone knows the layout of the building just a little better than I do. That it's not just someone. It's the kid who failed the class or got embarrassed or needed just the right thing said to him at just the right moment, and I missed that moment. Or, it's not even a former student, just another man struggling with entitlement and rage, with access to a weapon to which he shouldn't have access, just long enough for someone to say *hey, let's talk about mental health*, even though they have zero intention of even attempting to broach the subject and are only interested in the smoke screen, or in not having a conversation at all.

And it's not a sign of PTSD for my hands to go numb when the double doors unlock at the school entrance at 8:30 a.m. to let the kids file in. I just have to refocus. Be productive. Stay vigilant. Otherwise, I make small mistakes. Miss the stop sign. Forget the blinker. Don't quite have enough time between me and the police car to bring the speed down to something reasonable. And the last time I got pulled over I was too terrified to remember everything I'd been taught about what you're supposed to say to a policeman to insure you get to drive away. Is it hands on the steering wheel until they start asking questions or have your license and registration ready? Sob story or accountability? I have three apps on my phone designed to monitor these kinds of encounters, to record the audio and send it to a predetermined contact, but if I am too rattled to remember the rules my parents started teaching before I could barely ride a bike, I am certainly too rattled to drum up the name of an app I've not had to use once—which is when, I guess, I just take a deep breath and prepare to be another name on yet another protest sign.

Or maybe there is no protest. Because I am the type to be forgotten. And by forgotten, I mean Black and woman and queer, and therefore intentionally pushed to the side. And it's not a sign of anxiety anymore if the ruminations are based on reality. It is not a stretch to believe that, depending on the news coverage of the tragedy, mine will be on the list of names no one remembers, or even gets to hear in the first place. And if the whole of me will be deemed unremarkable anyway, why would I ever leave the bed?

It's not like the bed is all that safe anyway. How many times have Black homes been raided? Been moved? Flooded? Mistaken for a different home? Didn't we play *smear the queer* in school? Isn't that one of the places we're supposed to be safe? What is justice for a murdered woman when no one will admit that she is dead? Or even missing? Who decides if we're worthy of being found?

What I mean is, define *day-to-day life*. Is any of this how any of us are supposed to be living? Are we sure this is what we want to call normal? What I mean is, they used to call it a mental illness when enslaved people had the desire to escape—a more severe case if ever they tried to run away. And obviously I am not a slave, but I am still required to earn my keep here. To prove my worth inside the machine. Play my part and *earn a living*. And isn't that a telling phrase that we use to describe these jobs we do? That somehow, we must earn our right to be alive? By making a profit. For someone else. Who may or may not want to kill me. Or, at the very least has no vested interest in whether I stay alive. What I mean is, do I really have a disorder or an appropriate response to the conditions in which I am made to live? Am I depressed or just paying attention?

RESEARCH
(Erasure 4)

Scientists have ███████ discovered a single cause ████████████ Currently, they believe ████████████████████████

Genetics. ██
██
██
██

██

SESSION

FADE IN:

INT. ASHLEY'S OFFICE

Seated at her desk, logged into an early morning virtual therapy session with DR.THERAPY APP, a late forties Black woman. We can see both faces on ASHLEY's desktop computer. She appears exhausted.

> DR. THERAPY APP
> How are you feeling this morning?

> ASHLEY
> I'm ok.

> DR. THERAPY APP
> Ashley.

> ASHLEY
> I am. There was a moment this morning, but I was able to push through.

> DR. THERAPY APP
> Tell me more about the moment.

> ASHLEY
> Same old same.

> DR. THERAPY APP
> It seems as though you may be a little resistant to conversation this morning? Am I reading that correctly?

> ASHLEY
> Not resistant, per se. I just don't particularly want to talk about the obvious.

> DR. THERAPY APP
> Ok. What would you like to talk about?

> ASHLEY
> I mean. Obviously, I know what I need to talk about.

> DR. THERAPY APP
> It's not obvious to me. What do you want to talk about this morning?

                    ASHLEY
I don't know what there is to say.

                    DR. THERAPY APP
That's fair. Let's just start with the moment
from this morning. Give me two sentences that
are true.

                    ASHLEY
I had the dream again.

                    (Beat)

And there were tears.

                    DR. THERAPY APP
Ok. You had the dream, which we've been
anticipating. And we are not afraid of tears.
How was Cole?

                    ASHLEY
She let me have space to myself to cry. Made
me some tea.

                    DR. THERAPY APP
And how did that feel for you?

                    ASHLEY
Better than previous years, I guess. Felt like
she was trying her best to be supportive.

                    DR. THERAPY APP
Trying her best? Did you actually feel supported?

                    ASHLEY
She tried to push me out of bed too early.

                    DR. THERAPY APP
And how did you react to that?

                    ASHLEY
Not a total meltdown. But more tears.

                    DR. THERAPY APP
Were the tears a reaction to her pushing? Or
still a reaction to the dream?

                    ASHLEY
The dream, I think. Maybe both?

                    DR. THEARPY APP
Say more.

                    ASHLEY
It felt, maybe like she was checking boxes.
Like she'd done everything on her checklist
that she was supposed to do, and then when I
didn't react the way she'd hoped, she just
started getting pushy.

                    DR. THERAPY APP
Did she continue, as you said, to be pushy
when she saw that you were crying?

                    ASHLEY
No.

                    DR. THERAPY APP
What happened?

                    ASHLEY
She walked me through the thing.

                    DR. THERAPY APP
And did that help?

                    ASHLEY
Yes.

                    DR. THERAPY APP
Good. Let's go a little further into that. Did
you ask her to walk you through the exercise
or did she initiate?

                    ASHLEY
It was her.

                    DR. THERAPY APP
And did that feel pushy to you?

                    ASHLEY
No. That felt like the support I needed.

                    DR. THERAPY APP
And once you were calm?

                    ASHLEY
She made me breakfast. We started the day.

                    DR. THERAPY APP
Did that feel like checking boxes?

                    ASHLEY
Yes.

                    DR. THERAPY APP
But it helped?

                    ASHLEY
Yes.

                    DR. THERAPY APP
Ok. When you feel like she's just checking
boxes, how do you respond?

                    ASHLEY
I don't. There's nothing wrong with having
a checklist.

                    DR. THERAPY APP
As long as she doesn't get pushy about it.

                    ASHLEY
Right.

                    DR. THERAPY APP
Is it possible that you were trying to find
fault with her this morning so that you did not
have to focus on your own feelings of grief?

                    ASHLEY
Hey now. I thought we weren't talking about
the obvious.

                    DR. THERAPY APP
Is that obvious to you?

                    ASHLEY
No. I'm deflecting. Like a good patient.

                    DR. THERAPY APP
And you're using humor to stand apart from the
tension that you're feeling.

                    ASHLEY
Right on schedule.

                    DR. THERAPY APP
          Let's walk into that. You made the choice to
          schedule an extra session this week in order
          to process any feelings that might be coming
          up for you, yes?

                    ASHLEY
          Sure.

                    DR. THERAPY APP
          And you made the brave choice not to cancel.

                    ASHLEY
          Sure.

                    DR. THERAPY APP
          What were you hoping to explore when you
          logged on?

                    ASHLEY
          I don't know. Maybe I wanted to tell you a few jokes.

                    DR. THERAPY APP
          Don't take the cop out. You had some expectation
          for what you might need to explore today. Think
          it through.

                    ASHLEY
          I wanted to talk about the dream.

                    DR. THERAPY APP
          Yes. This dream. That happens like clockwork.
          Every year. The night before the anniversary.

                    ASHLEY
          Not the same way each time, though.

                    DR. THERAPY APP
          What was the major difference this year?

                    ASHLEY
          She opened her eyes.

                    DR. THERAPY APP
          And did you have some awareness in the dream
          of what that meant?

                    ASHLEY
          Yes.

                    DR. THERAPY APP

                       (Beat)

What did it mean?

                       ASHLEY
That she's still alive.

                    DR. THERAPY APP
Is that perhaps why your reaction was so raw
this morning? To wake up and realize that
she wasn't?

                       ASHLEY
That's not what I realized.

                    DR. THERAPY APP
Push.

                       ASHLEY
It was like. I can only see her in my dreams.

                    DR. THERAPY APP
Was that a difficult realization to come to?

                       ASHLEY
No.

                    DR. THERAPY APP
What else?

                       ASHLEY
It's the only time I can see her.

                    DR. THERAPY APP
Push.

                       ASHLEY

                       (Beat)

I really want the dreams to stop.

DR. THERAPY APP sits back in her chair, smiling. It is clear she
feels this is the beginning of a breakthrough. ASHLEY shuffles papers
on her desk, then pulls up the Messenger app on her computer. The
text to Cole reads *"How much longer do I have to stay on this Zoom?"*

                                              FADE OUT.

UNTITLED

every shirt folded
every sock paired
each carpet vacuumed
every bed made
every sink wiped
every dish washed
every book shelved
every lamp dusted
all the trash bagged
each letter written
every pill swallowed
done with spring cleaning

If perhaps you are foolish enough to follow your coworkers on social media, there are moments when you are expected to share a few photos. Spring Break. Thanksgiving. The first few days of summer. But the languishing week between Christmas and New Year? Middle of July? Memorial Day weekend? These are generous pockets of time where no one expects to see you—long stretches where most people forget teachers even exist. So, of course, it's a good time to kill yourself. Because no one is going to check on you. A teacher with the time management skills the profession requires can be dead enough for a closed casket funeral long before anyone knows you are gone, even with a day or two at the top to write letters and tidy affairs.

The options will feel almost endless. Unless, of course, you are still keeping that promise about not going out with a razor blade, even though the person to whom you made the promise doesn't answer your calls anymore—something about codependence and being the reason they too are now depressed. And of course, you are opposed to gun violence—even inflicted upon yourself; too scared for heights; too in love with your car to let it be your carriage to the astral plane—which of course, leaves only pills, though they have let you down every time you have tried. Years ago, before the diagnosis—sleep deprived after nearly six straight hours in prayer—after seeing the face of a terrifying god who told you *No* yet again. And then, years after, when you decided that same *No* could come from your own hands.

Waking up at home after a failed attempt is the worst kind of waking.

To begin, you are in pain. Knotted stomach. Screaming head. Sometimes, but not always, covered in your own sick. And then. You are in pain. All of your reasons from the night before come flooding back into the room, and now, wading into those waters is the fact that you are bad at dying—which any idiot should just be able to do.

There are three viable options:

Obviously. Try again. Immediately. Leave no time to think things through. Except, if you have already tried your best, there are no more pills for you to take, and even the empty bottles are judging you with an exhausted disdain.

Or. You can phone a friend, a neighbor, maybe one of those coworkers. Put a vague post on Facebook and hope for the best. But the best, is honestly a *5150*, which is decidedly out of the question. The whole point was to die with no one the wiser. Getting committed will require taking sick days, and no one wants to waste a sick day on actually being unwell. And what will a friend who won't have you committed be able to do beyond notice all of the things that are wrong with you when you are already so painfully aware.

Which leaves only sleep. Hope the drugs need more time to work. That the knot in your stomach is a time released capsule that won't let you down if you manage to crawl from the bathroom floor to the couch—maybe guzzle down whatever remains from whatever bottles are in the freezer and slowly allow yourself to drift into a godless haze.

The great thing about return to school platitudes is that no one really cares what you did over the break. It's like the question, *How are you doing?* You could say: *"My heart is a bottomless ocean full of creatures no one has discovered yet, but the ones we do have names for are so ghastly we are terrified to gaze upon them. Some day, I think I will drown there. It is so cold, and I'm running out of air."* But instead, you say, *"Pretty good, how are you,"* then nod along to whatever lie your conversation partner tells.

It's easy. You say, *"What did you do over break?"* They respond, *"Graded papers. Read a novel. Watched a little TV."* You say, *"Oh! What did I do? Nothing much. Kinda rested. Got a lot of sleep."*

CANTOR WRITES A SUICIDE NOTE
THEN TOSSES IT INTO THE SNOW

There is a difference between the countably infinite
and that which is uncountable:
The rain that falls to water the earth / the vapor to which it distills.

My students say the thing about always adding one.
I ask if there is nothing smaller worthy of addition.

There is an infinite number of numbers between zero and one.
Some of them we have names for / others are just a thought.

I am alive today because an old friend thought of me once—
Reminded me of promises made a third of our lives ago.

She asks me to name one thing worth enduring any storm,
Then watches me distill that thing down to its vapor.

My brother / becomes his laughter / becomes the air between his teeth.
There is a countable number of atoms there but no way for me to count them.
She asks if I will keep breathing to honor molecules too small to see.

A student trips in the hallway / another says go kill yourself.
Everyone around the two of them laughs, even the one who's the butt of the joke

I hear the laughter fall to the ground / the sadness to which it distills.
There is a countable number of suicide attempts of high school students this year
An uncountable number of times they've smiled while sharpening the blade

I am alive today because a teacher saw an off-kilter grin once Asked me to
dream of a future with too many joys to count.

My student who slipped me a suicide note the third day of his sophomore
year walks across the graduation stage and I know that dream is here

Depression is a countable weight / the days can feel so uncountable An uncountable number of moments between each one and the next

It is an insatiable river held back by a levee I built myself.
A countable number of times it's broken with no time to prepare.

I am alive today because I decided to get out of bed once.
Decided to eat / decided to shower / decided to live up to my own good name

Each night the darkness threatens I promise myself I will add another day
And know it only comes with moment-by-moment addition.

There are days I am drowned in sorrow and the guilt that it distills to—
Days I cannot see the difference between the rain and all this vapor.

I am alive / I am alive / I am alive / I am alive
I am built to withstand the water.
I declare my own name at the mouth of the river.

It does not matter how many atoms comprise every storm.
This rain is not infinite / vapor not infinite
Depression not infinite
I am.

A THEOLOGY OF
MANIC DEPRESSION

1   The search for absolute truth must begin before the symptoms.
     Anything that comes after may be fodder for the break.

2   God exists. And loves you.

     You believe this most of the time—enough to say it out loud
     to other people. Sometimes while standing behind a pulpit.

     All of this from before.

     All of this certainly true.

3   All the prophets were street performers. Noah built a boat
     and warned the people of drowning, even though they'd
     never seen or heard of rain. Ezekiel travelled, naked and
     barefoot, laying siege to miniature models of the temple.
     Elijah—performance art with fire. John the Baptizer wore
     elaborate costumes and sometimes did strange things with
     his food. And all you are is a poet. Sometimes on a street
     corner. Most of the time from a well-lit stage. Strangers are
     compelled to hear what you say.

     You must be like one of the prophets. Not crazy. Not sick.
     Not what they say. Something like sacred at your core—you
     speak on behalf of god.

4   God does not speak to people like you.

     You vessel of dishonor.

     Reprobate thing.

     Hell now or later.

     Suffering inevitable.

     You may as well be dead.

5   Every prayer journal you've not thrown away has one thing
    in common: A page a little further back than the middle,
    just before you abandon it for a better notebook, tear or
    wine-stained in tiny enough handwriting for god to read it
    as a whisper. Your heart broken. Your soul tired. Just one
    word: *Please*.

6   A psychotic break is a kind of vision.

    Your mind eager for the hallucination.

    A hospital can become a temple.

    The doctors lead the call to worship.

    Call every patient here a member of your congregation.

7   What is the line of demarcation between hearing from god or
    some other, less acceptable voice? Is it spiritual? Chemical?
    Audience driven? One you tell your therapist? The other
    anyone who will listen?

8   And now that you have seen the light, you will build a group
    of new believers. Following Jesus. Reading the ancients.
    Bible. Quran. Book of the Dead. Euclid's *Axioms*—all of it
    useful. We will come to know the absolute truth. Every holy
    book. Every god.

9   Haven't you heard?

    I am your god.

10 Mental illness in the Bible is characterized by demon
    possession—the kind that brings with it seizures or self-
    harm. Are you an embodied evil? Are you a cursed soul?

11 I am the voice crying out in the wilderness. Prepare ye the
    way of the Lord.

12   And Khadijah said: *Never! By Allah, He would not disgrace you
      with madness,* as Mohammed lay weeping after leaving the cave.

13   What is true?

      God loves you. Most of the time.

      You believe this enough to say it aloud in the mirror on the
      days you feel like he does not.

14   You will write your own holy book.

15   *Please*

      Please

      Please

Stages are good. Pulpits are good. Anywhere with a platform and a microphone is good. Crowds are bad. Crowds are volatile. Audiences are good. Audiences can be held in the palm of one's hand. A class is a captive audience. A lesson plan is a performance. Performance is good. Teaching is good. A classroom is a sanctuary.

I began my teaching career in August 2008, a few weeks after resolving what my second doctor later labelled my first full manic episode. I was broke, exhausted, demoralized, and terrified—exactly like every other first year teacher in the building. We swapped "last summer of freedom" stories in the teachers' lounge over lunch during those initial workdays. A few read *The First Days of School* with highlighters at the ready. A few spoke of day trips with grad school friends.

The teachers' lounge is good. Openness with new friends is good. Admitting near-reckless impulsivity to strangers who are now coworkers is bad. I was an island to myself that first year. Most of my dedication to teaching was born in that lounge for no other reason than proving I was sane enough to do it. To them. To myself.

I think a lot about what went wrong that year—all the places where I can place blame. I wasn't a horrible teacher, but I was nowhere near as good as I thought I was, either. But a first-year teacher on the downswing of mania is hesitant to show any fear. She does not need to ask questions. She doesn't need any help. And of course, even if I did need help, it felt mostly unattainable. My mentor teacher under whom I'd apprenticed was dealing with the loss of a parent; between her own classroom, grief, and handling family affairs, she had little time or space to attend to my teaching practice—not that I would have heeded any of her advice.

But. A first year with a lot to prove does not need actual mentoring, nor unpacked standards or access to the curriculum pacing guide. She can shoulder the weight of 120 eighth graders with a couple of years old teachers' editions, while also being an ear to incomparable grief. Being present is good.

67

Overconfidence is bad. Having a scapegoat at the ready was comforting just in case the crazy reared its head.

And it did. A little. The thing with the calculators. An almost compulsive need to hoard them. To have thirty-six on hand at all times, even though my largest class was only thirty-two. I counted them before and after each class—made students turn in phones or necklaces or their lunchboxes as collateral—developed increasingly elaborate systems for making sure I always had enough. I stored them in a bin in my filing cabinet, away from the prying eyes of administrators who asked us daily to watch the students who were clearly pilfering the school's supply.

Hearing students consistently accused of theft did not compel me to divulge my shameful secret. It barely registered as a real concern amidst the ever-growing list of my students' struggles: students who could barely handle addition, much less the algebra I was expected to teach them; students who couldn't be counted on to regularly attend school. Even these very real (though commonplace) problems paled in comparison to the painful stories somehow my first-year group of students trusted me to hold: stories of self-harm and questions about coming out of the closet, heartbreaking tales about going hungry and parents that did not come home. All of this weighed on me more and more heavily—made it more necessary for me to show that I could teach them, despite all the dark we shared.

Our shortage of calculators though, would eventually interfere with my ability to prove myself. Without turning them in to be properly cleared, we could not administer the mandatory testing. Our curriculum coordinator cried in my classroom after being reprimanded by our tyrant principal; apparently the burden of providing calculators rested squarely on her shoulders. She did not understand where the last forty or so had gone. I let her cry. Gave reassurances. Did not let on where the calculators had been.

It was in fact that testing that finally bore out my secret. After each of three district tests, we were allowed a window of a few weeks to review the results with our students. Our curriculum coordinator created elaborate spreadsheets detailing which groups of students should review which groups of questions. I kept the spreadsheets and all the test materials in haphazard piles on the side of my desk. Each day we worked through a few of the problems. I pulled the test books mostly at random and threw them back into the piles. Then, on the last day we were allowed to keep them, I somehow only brought back thirty-one books for a class of thirty-two. And maybe it wasn't the felony I was told it was, but it was in fact a fireable offense—failing to return all test materials—an infraction for which my teaching license could be suspended and ultimately revoked altogether.

We counted and recounted each of the books. Answer sheets. Even the scratch paper. Again and again, and then I was grilled. Where could they be? Exactly in my classroom. I was told to offer up all the locations my testing materials had ever been held. Desk. Closet. Filing cabinet. And then for some reason, I was made to remain in the office, banned from my classroom, until the administration was able to recover the missing student book.

A messy desk is good. Finding the test there is good. Finding it after the curriculum coordinator looks in the filing cabinet is devastating. How to explain that I understood her frustration, but she still can't possibly take the calculators away? Doesn't matter that fewer than half of them have ever seen the light of day. Doesn't matter that most of your students barely know how to turn them on.

The letter for my file mentioned reckless disregard for the handling of school property and personnel, which felt laughable at best, but I did not laugh as my tyrant principal droned on from his chair. His assistant scribbled down what he was saying on a fresh yellow legal pad, subtly shaking her head *"no"* every time she saw me about to lean in and interject. I found the idea of enduring his rant in silence even less humorous than being made to sit there at all, until later, when a card for our unofficial union made its way to the corner of my slightly less messy desk. They listened to, and in a later meeting, reiterated all of my questions: *What supports are being provided for other first year teachers? Do you even have mentorship program? At the very least, shouldn't every math teacher have a class set of the calculators their students will need to pass a mandatory test? A test that is so important that misplaced materials are worthy of losing a job?*

Self-preservation is good. Denial is good. A tyrant can become a captive audience. Performance is good. Seeing a letter shredded is good. A locked file cabinet is a sanctuary.

No one says *suicidal ideation* when you decide to get a cat. The people closest to you wonder how you will keep the thing alive; how you'll keep the apartment clean; judge you silently for the obvious stereotypes—but they don't think *death wish* immediately. And the cat is...good. A quiet little rescue, cuddly and kind of stupid—wants to be an outdoor cat but is terrified by everything. The poet in you is thrilled by the metaphor, but there's still a litter box and that is disgusting. Miraculously though, the cat is a neat freak and reminds you to clean more often than you'd like to, especially on the days she has to claw you out of bed. And she has to eat, so you have to go shopping; you take regular showers because she likes the steam. In so many small ways that no one could have predicted, this cat is an answer to your friends' prayers—even when they had so much doubt.

Except. You are allergic. Which you knew before you got her. So, you prepped by stocking up on homeopathic allergy pills; refilled the prescription for your steroid inhaler; chose not to take both at the recommended intervals, and suffered through whenever she sits on your lap. Two or so years later, you change apartments (slash hastily move in with another girl who's more depressed than you), but the cat cannot go with you. Re-homing is a sad, yet guiltless process, and slowly, it becomes easier to breathe.

This is what it is to not want to die, while embracing the casually reckless. The pack-and-a-half a day smoking habit. Going every other day on the medications. Taking late and long enough drives so you drift off to sleep or are forced to spend the night in your car. And you aren't allowed to say this out loud, but sometimes you envy those of your friends who took more decisive actions—none of this slow-motion-god-get-me-out-of-here-leave-it-to-chance nonsense that you are relying on to be your way of escape.

Perhaps *casual* isn't the word. Well-intentioned. Even a gift. Because you know your friends are praying. When you send them a text at 4 a.m., or call but can't eke out a single word. They pray that something they say will pull you back from the edge. That this time the saying actually sticks and the edge will soften or disappear. That deep down they are counting down the days until they get the call they know is someday coming. But wouldn't this be more refreshing? An accident? Unexpected tragedy? Even something silly like the wrong antihistamine when the second cat arrives after you've found a different place to stay?

In almost all the self help books you read they mention the power of repeated small actions. Wake up at 6 long enough, and eventually you'll make it on time to work. Drive 30 or so over the speed limit without enough sleep and eventually the guardrail will find you.

And that doesn't count as by your own hand. And won't that be a relief?

SYNDICATION

There are only so many times you can quit your job and burn through your very meager savings, especially if you do very little to replenish them before quitting your job again—so every time you do, it must be for a spectacular reason, not something as frivolous as impressing a pretty girl with the way you are able to operate with no strings attached, but if somehow you can pull that off too, it is a nice cherry on top—and after all, you do have a type.

Gorgeous, of course. With dreams of independence. Fresh out of the kind of relationship that makes them afraid to look in the mirror, with a basket of red flags almost as large as your own that you pull out in handfuls to wave at each other like matadors desperately trying not to see each other's bull.

We met at a

writers' workshop

tent revival

cocktail party

poetry slam.

And the whole room faded away to a cinematic nothing. You are good at making someone the absolute center of your attention until they feel as if they're the only person that's ever mattered in your world. You ask

what kind of pen they prefer

their favorite scripture

to buy them a drink.

And the conversation doesn't feel prescriptive, even though it very much is. Even this, your first interaction, like a movie you've seen several times before. You ask

What brings you here?

And lean into a mundane response

Just trying to get better

Love this preacher

Got invited by work friends

Love to listen to poems

You say, *"No. What brought you here? What did you hope would happen? Why are you here with me?"* Then you wait for the broken wing. We bonded over

A love of language

Religious trauma

Too many shots to be remembered the next day

A hastily written poem

Some stereotypes are vile exaggerations if not outright lies; others, unfortunately are true. You declare your love in

ten days

about a month

seventy-two hours

And your friends don't hear from you for weeks, not really. The occasional text message or Facebook post. You are deep in the trenches of your brand-new love—the one who is different from all the others. The one you can see for how incredible they are despite

the abusive ex

neglectful parents

fear of failure

and you are just the person to lead them back to themselves. You're on the verge of changing the world anyway. With your latest project. Latest plan. And they get to be by your side for all of it, plus the road trip, lake house, restaurant opening—the small town glam of you throwing it away—day by day like a death march that feels like a great time. Somewhere between three and six months

you move in with her

she moves in with you

You are stringing together micro part-time jobs and start hinting at marriage. You can see the future so clearly—moments away from your big break with the right girl beside you, even if she keeps suggesting it might be time to see a doctor for the insomnia and struggling speech. And she doesn't mean to nag about how you don't help out around the apartment, or even get out of bed to do much of anything these days. Or how you're not making good on the promises you made what feels like not that long ago. Even though none of that matters. After all, you were the one that saved her and are owed at the very least an acquiescent devotion. Because it's never been this bad before. And you know you can get better. And you will blow it apart yourself before admitting you are unworthy of worship. You fight. Call on every insecurity. You lie. You cheat.

You leave

You leave

You leave

You leave

There are only so many times you can somehow pretend to be the good guy in every story. Even if the plot never changes. And you can already see the end.

And obviously you should tell your mother. She'll worry. Or maybe not know how to take it, but at the very least she will know. Your brother knows. Not anything so stark as the official diagnosis, but in that weird way he always knows when something is going on with you long before you confess. And you are not ready to confess, no matter the good it's supposed to do. Bringing the whole family in is supposedly a part of getting better—healing the traumas that could have been symptoms; having a support team, a crisis plan in place. And what if you can actually pray away the crazy? Not you obviously, but you were in the room that one time she prayed for your friend that had the grotesque knot protruding from her leg, and you watched it shrink into nothing while everyone around her shouted and cried, so if anyone could convince god to cut you a break it would definitely have to be your mother, even if you're not entirely convinced that wasn't a hallucination too. Though you do believe in miracles.

How else do you explain how you are still here despite your best efforts not to be? How else to explain the breath in your lungs except for the fact that your mother prays? And doesn't that, at the very least, earn her the right to know?

You do talk every Sunday. About a million little things. Your students. Her doctors' appointments. Dinner plans. Church. It's a masterful volley—a form of protection you've been perfecting for almost as long as you can remember. Like decades ago when you were a child and convinced her that you didn't actually want to get braces to save her from the hushed conversations you overhead about their expense. Or years later, when you weaved a masterful tale about losing the trail in the woods near your house when she saw your arms and her face asked the question she couldn't quite verbalize.

But what would you even say at this point? After so many years of lying? After so many years of hiding the sad, Sunday after Sunday? Of sending a text instead of calling on the days you were swallowed up by the sheets? Saying you're sick? Or exhausted? Will try again the next day? All these not-quite lies when you couldn't keep the tears out of your voice.

And if you tell your mother, you will then actually be bipolar, no matter what you tell your friends about the sinister futility of labels, and of all the so-called identities you have taught yourself to be ok with holding. Bipolar is the one thing these days you do not want to be. It feels like a death sentence. Feels like you are not in control. Feels like the only thing that will matter once everyone knows.

You are terrified of terrifying your mother. If she knows you cannot protect her. She will know that every time the phone goes to voicemail on a Sunday when you are supposed to connect, it was because you couldn't confine yourself to the small talk. Pop's latest gadgets. The book you're reading. Your niece's brilliance. Church again. Simply could not pick up the phone because all you had to say was goodbye, and what kind of thing is that to say to your mother from all those miles away?

You are terrified she won't be terrified. Just shocked into action. If she knows you cannot protect yourself. She will hop on a one-way ticket with anointing oil and open arms. And there is something grotesque here, but you already feel small enough to be nothing.

288   Under His Wings   TRUST

Words: William Orcutt Cushing, 1896.
Music and Setting: 'Under His Wings' Ira David Sankey, 1898.

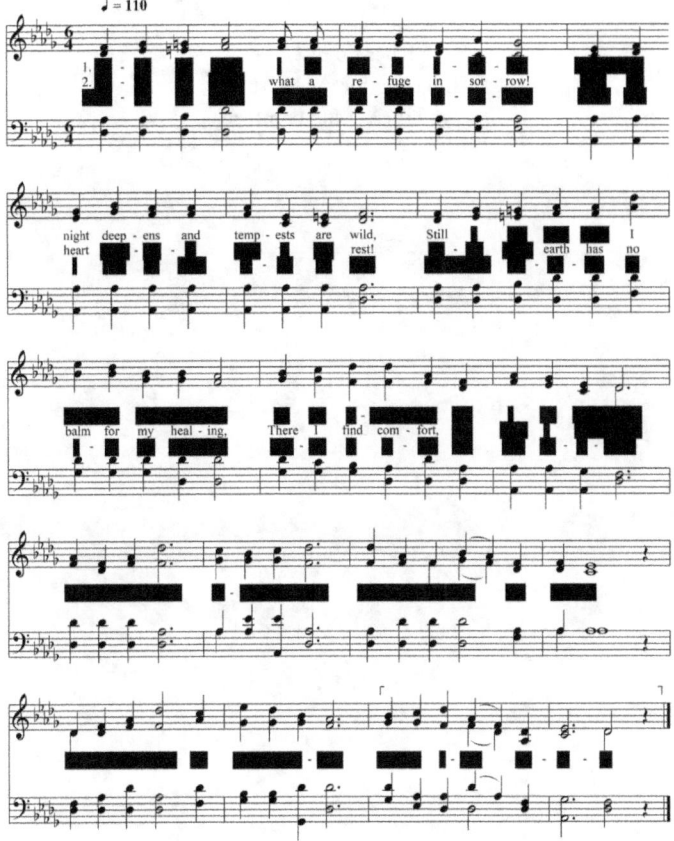

Ps 17:7-9, Mt 11:28   11 10 11 10 8 7 9 7

the night deepens
and tempests are wild
still i refuge in sorrow

earth has no rest
no balm for my heart
still there i find comfort

CLIENT INTAKE FORM

This form is used to collect information about new clients and is for internal purposes only. The information you provide is confidential and will be treated accordingly.

REASONS FOR VISIT

What are the problems for which you are seeking help?

Med Check

Current Symptoms: (check all that apply)

☐ Racing thoughts	☐ Fatigue	☐ Excessive energy	☒ Depressed mood
☐ Suspiciousness	☐ Hallucinations	☐ Impulsivity	☒ Loss of interest
☐ Avoidance	☐ Forgetfulness	☐ Change in appetite	☐ Crying spell
☐ Anxiety Attacks	☐ Excessive Guilt	☐ Excessive worry	☐ Increased irritiability
☐ Sleep pattern disturbance	☐ Unable to enjoy activities	☐ Increased risky behavior	☐ Decreased need for sleep

June 2017

CLIENT INTAKE FORM

This form is used to collect information about new clients and is for internal purposes only. The information you provide is confidential and will be treated accordingly.

REASONS FOR VISIT

What are the problems for which you are seeking help?

Med Check

Current Symptoms: (check all that apply)

☐ Racing thoughts	☐ Fatigue	☐ Excessive energy	☒ Depressed mood
☐ Suspiciousness	☐ Hallucinations	☐ Impulsivity	☒ Loss of interest
☒ Avoidance	☐ Forgetfulness	☐ Change in appetite	☐ Crying spell
☐ Anxiety Attacks	☐ Excessive Guilt	☐ Excessive worry	☐ Increased irritiability
☐ Sleep pattern disturbance	☐ Unable to enjoy activities	☐ Increased risky behavior	☐ Decreased need for sleep

June 2018

BLOOD TEST: REPRISE

FADE IN:

EXT. CITY PARK—MID AFTERNOON

It's a cold, winter day.

ASHLEY, now in her early 30's, lies on her back on a park bench, staring into a gray sky. She has just left a session with her therapist, the office visible in the background. She is noticeably underdressed for the weather as compared to *RENEE*, seated on the bench beside her.

> RENEE
> So what…you're just better now?

> ASHLEY
> She didn't say better.

> RENEE
> She said…

> ASHLEY
> That at this point in managing my illness, statistically I can expect to remain, I guess, even.

> RENEE
> So, like. You're possibly better.

> ASHLEY
> Probably. Asymptomatic.

> RENEE
> For…

> ASHLEY
> The foreseeable future, I guess.

> RENEE
> You guess.

> ASHLEY
> I think she guesses too.

                         RENEE
          I don't know how I should respond to that.

*Renee pulls her phone from her pocket, removes a glove, and begins
to type. We do not see the screen of her phone. The two sit for a
few moments in silence.*

                         RENEE
          Is there a more definitive test you can take?

                         ASHLEY
          Like on Buzzfeed?

                         RENEE
          Like the thing with the butterflies. Or maybe
          a blood test or something

                         ASHLEY
          I've done all the questionnaires a million
          times. I think I'd have more luck with Buzzfeed.

                    (Beat)

          I think this is supposed to be the good news part.

                         RENEE
          Probably.

                         ASHLEY
          Yes. With great odds. You could stop waiting
          for the other shoe to drop every time I tell
          you that I have an idea about something. Is this
          brilliance? Is this mania? You'd already know.
          You'd finally have to come around to my genius.

                         RENEE
          And we're already back to delusions of grandeur.

                         ASHLEY
          No delusions. Just grand.

                         RENEE
          And not really even, right? It's just the mania?

                         ASHLEY
          Apparently the sad still stays.

                    (Beat)

          Not as bad though. Less severe. Less often.

                    RENEE
          Possibly.

                    ASHLEY
          Do we need to have a conversation about
          the difference between probability and its
          lesser twin?

                    RENEE
          Stop trying to argue the semantics. I'm trying
          to have a conversation about how this doesn't
          feel like good news.

                    ASHLEY
          I know.

Ashley sits upright.

                    ASHLEY
          Remember that time I went catatonic, and you
          thought I was having a stroke, but really I
          was just so sleep deprived that my body could
          literally no longer function? Got to the
          hospital, got a little sedation so I could
          finally catch some z's?

                    RENEE
          Of course I remember. I was terrified. You're the
          one who doesn't actually remember—woke up like
          you were just finishing a twenty-minute nap.

                    ASHLEY
          I'm saying. No more of that. That has to at
          least count for something.

                    RENEE
          It does. It would just count for more if we
          had a little certainty.

                    ASHLEY
          I am certain.

                    RENEE
          Weren't you just talking to me about probabilities?

                    ASHLEY
          Hey now. I'm the mathematician. You should
          trust me when I say I am certain.

                    RENEE
About what part?

                    ASHLEY
That the worst of it's over.

                    RENEE
Yeah, and if not?

                    ASHLEY
I'll keep fighting. Find my way back.

                                        FADE OUT.

ASHLEY LUMPKIN is a Georgia-raised, Carolina-based writer, editor, actor, and educator. She is the author of five poetry collections: {} At First Sight, Second Glance, Terrorism and Other Topics for Tea, #AshleyLumpkin, and Genesis. Her book, I Hate You All Equally, is a collection of conversations from her years as a classroom teacher.

A lover of performance as well as the written word, she has been a competing member of the Bull City Slam Team since 2015 and currently serves as its coach.

Above all else, Ashley considers herself a teacher, poet, and fryer of food. She is a lover of mathematics and language. She loves you too.

First printing
ISBN   978-1-95910-402-5

EDITORIAL AND DESIGN. Edited by Steve Mitchell. Editorial Assistance by Sarah Rhu. Cover and interior design by Andrew Saulters. Scuppernong Editions colophon by Rachel York.

TYPE. Titles and folios in Folio. Title page and cover in Goudy Old Style. Body text in Arno Pro and Folio.

Scuppernong Editions offers the occasional publication of adventuresome, commercially questionable writing in all genres.

Scuppernong Editions
304 South Elm Street
Greensboro, NC 27401